H is for Hockey

An NHL Alumni Alphabet

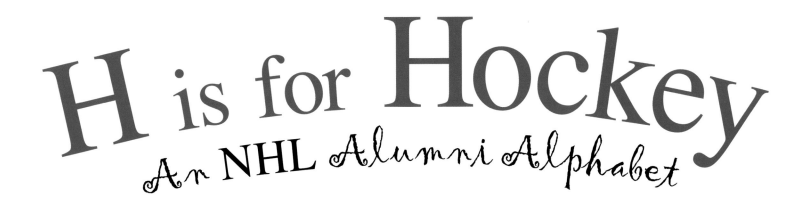

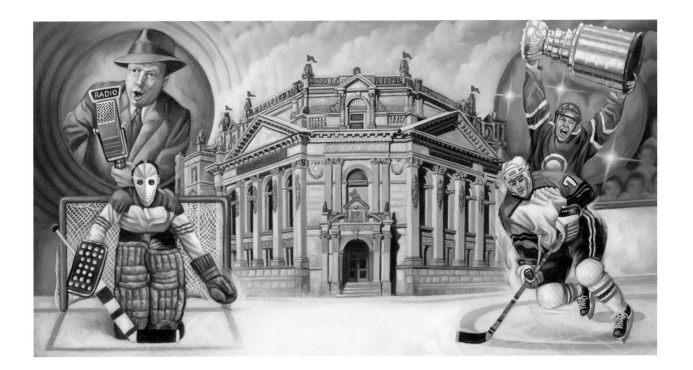

Written by Kevin Shea and Illustrated by Ken Dewar

This book is dedicated to the dreams of children everywhere.
Kevin

X

Of all the gifts that I have received in life—some luck, some talent—the greatest gift has been my family. For my mother Ethel Dewar (1926–2011)—"Cheers for now."
Ken

Sleeping Bear Press™
315 E. Eisenhower Parkway, Ste. 200
Ann Arbor, MI 48108
www.sleepingbearpress.com

Sleeping Bear Press, a part of Cengage Learning.

Printed and bound in the United States.

10 9 8 7 6 5 4 3 2 1

Library of Congress Cataloging-in-Publication Data

Shea, Kevin, 1956-
H is for hockey : an NHL alumni alphabet / written by Kevin Shea;
illustrated by Ken Dewar.
p. cm.
ISBN 978-1-58536-794-8 — ISBN 978-1-58536-814-3 (custom edition)
1. Hockey—Juvenile literature. I. Dewar, Ken, 1960- ill. II. Title.
GV847.25.S45 2012
796.962—dc23
2011052716

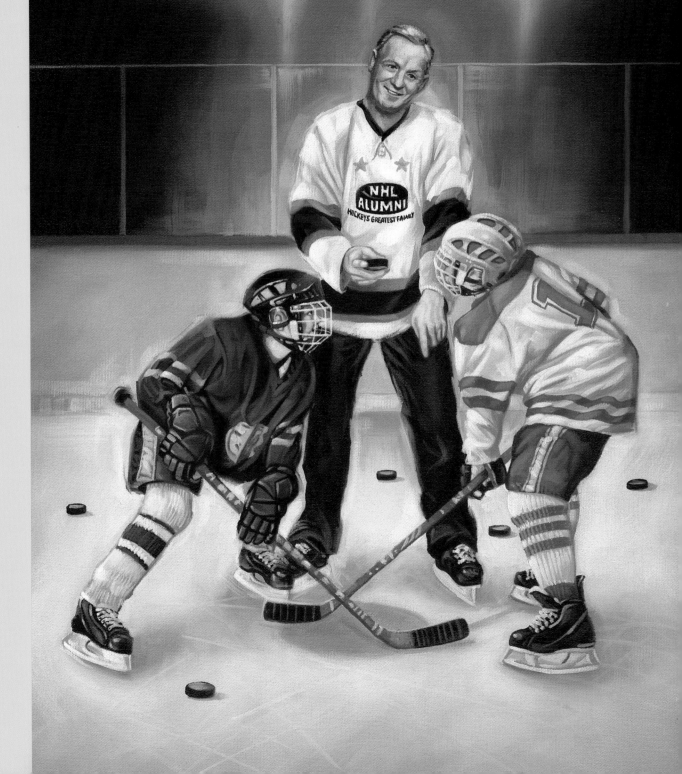

A is for Alumni,
who loved to play the game.
Fans cheered them on
and asked, "Please sign your name?"

Just over 5,000 players have played at least one game in the National Hockey League (NHL) since the league was formed in 1917. Affectionately known as "Hockey's Greatest Family," the NHL Alumni Association was established in 1999 and is based in Toronto, Ontario.

The organization's mission statement is: *The National Hockey League Alumni brings together former NHL players to support and participate in charitable causes, primarily those youth oriented; assist former players in their transition to life after hockey; promote the game of hockey.*

Fans will regularly see members of the NHL Alumni at a number of events, including hockey games, golf tournaments, speaking engagements, and autograph sessions. The money raised, which is more than one million dollars annually, goes to various causes, including scholarships and charities.

Many players, who have devoted their entire lives to playing hockey, are given a new start through the NHL Alumni Association once their NHL playing careers have come to an end.

Members of the Alumni Association are considered ambassadors of the history and tradition of the great game of hockey.

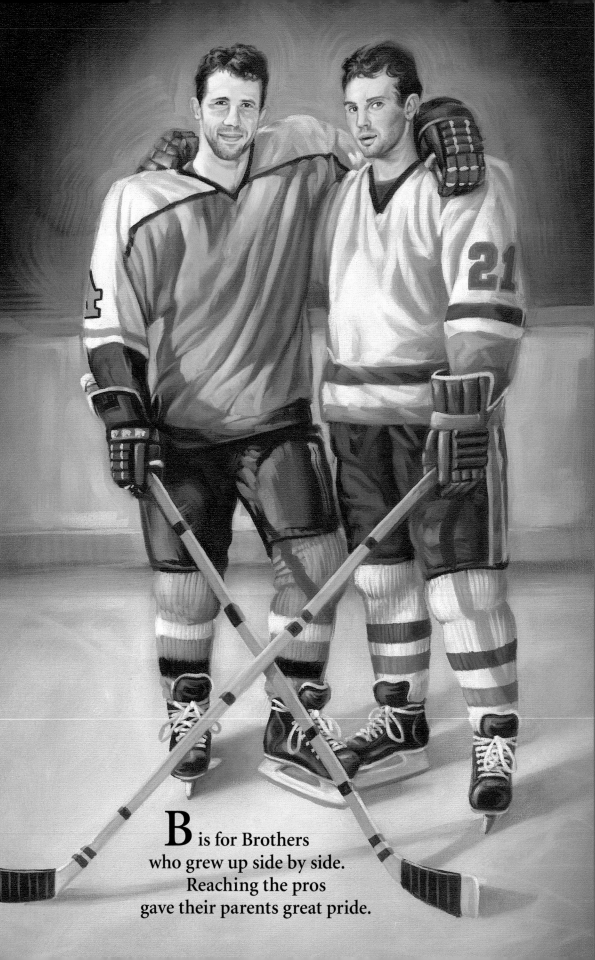

B is for Brothers
who grew up side by side.
Reaching the pros
gave their parents great pride.

There have been many brothers who have played in the NHL. The most well-known brothers might very well be Maurice and Henri Richard, who played for the Montreal Canadiens. Maurice won eight Stanley Cup championships and Henri won eleven. Another set of brothers is Lionel, Charlie, and Roy Conacher, all three of whom have been inducted into the Hockey Hall of Fame.

But no family has sent more brothers to the NHL than the Sutter family from Viking, Alberta. Brent, Brian, Darryl, Duane, Rich, and Ron collectively played more than 5,000 games in the NHL.

Several NHL superstars have had brothers who also played in the league. These include Wayne and Brent Gretzky, Gordie and Vic Howe, Mario and Alain Lemieux as well as Patrick and Stephane Roy.

B b

C stands for Canada,
    where hockey got its start,
and now it's a game
    that fills every fan's heart.

There is a great deal of discussion as to where the game of hockey was actually first played. There are some who claim that hockey was first played by Canadian troops on the frozen lakes around Halifax, Nova Scotia. Others swear the game was first played by students from King's College School on Long Pond, which is located on a pumpkin farm in Windsor, Nova Scotia. Still others believe that Sir John Franklin played hockey with his crew on Great Bear Lake during one of their Arctic expeditions. What we do know is that the very first organized indoor hockey game took place on March 3, 1875, at the Victoria Skating Rink in Montreal, Quebec.

Hockey is Canada's national winter sport. The game may have been born in Canada, but it is now played in countries around the globe. NHL players have come from such non-traditional hockey countries as Brazil (Robyn Regehr), Japan (Yutaka Fukufuji), Nigeria (Rumun Ndur), South Africa (Olaf Kölzig), and Tanzania (Chris Nielsen).

Dd

Dreaming of the Draft—
this brings us to D.
One boy goes each round.
Who will the next choice be?

The very first NHL draft took place in 1963, and only 11 players were selected. Before that, the six existing NHL teams were free to sign any players over the age of 13 who were not already under contract to another NHL team.

Today, each of the 30 NHL teams has the opportunity to draft one player in each of seven rounds. That means that every June, 210 young players realize a dream when they hear their name called by one of the 30 NHL teams.

When 17-year-old Sidney Crosby was drafted by the Pittsburgh Penguins in 2005, he said, "This is amazing. It's been a lot of hard work and a lot of sacrifices. It's unbelievable!"

Many good players, like Ed Belfour and Brian Rafalski, were never drafted but went on to outstanding NHL careers.

Most of us held our own "drafts" when we chose teams to play road hockey or "shinny." Sometimes, two captains would take turns choosing players for their teams. Other times, everyone's stick was randomly tossed into a pile, and the two captains would take turns tossing sticks onto their side. The players who belonged to those sticks became a team.

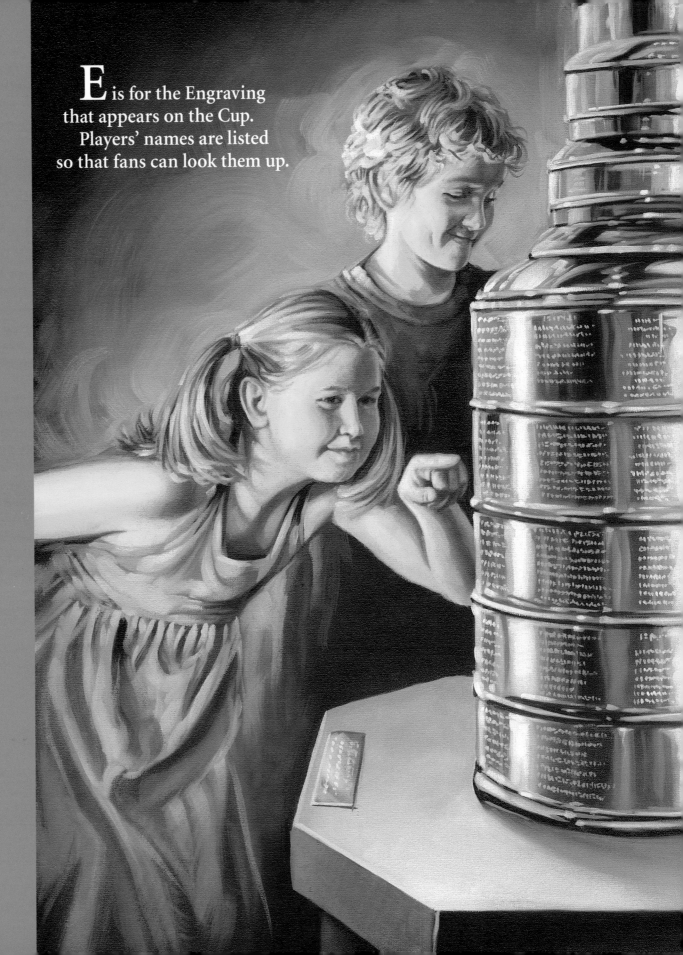

Each September, the Stanley Cup is taken to Montreal where the names of the new Stanley Cup champions are engraved onto hockey's greatest trophy.

The tradition began when the Montreal Wanderers won the Stanley Cup in 1907 and had the names of their players engraved inside the bowl of the Cup. Engraving the names of Stanley Cup winners became an annual tradition in 1924.

Currently, each Stanley Cup–winning team is allowed to have 52 names added to the trophy. Each name takes approximately 30 minutes to engrave using a small hammer and individual letters that are "punched" into the silver of the Cup. The engraver is given a week to engrave all the names.

To see their names engraved on the Stanley Cup along with the greats of the game—Maurice Richard, Gordie Howe, Bobby Orr, Wayne Gretzky, Steve Yzerman—is very emotional for the winning players.

The engravers occasionally make mistakes. The 1951–52 Detroit Red Wings have two errors on the Stanley Cup: Tommy Ivan, the coach, is misspelled as "Nivan" and Alex Delvecchio is incorrectly engraved as "Belvecchio." Poor Jacques Plante of the Montreal Canadiens was the goaltender on five consecutive Stanley Cup champions, but his name is spelled differently each year. The New York Islanders were surprised to see the team name spelled "Ilanders" in 1980–81.

E e

E is for the Engraving that appears on the Cup. Players' names are listed so that fans can look them up.

We cheer and we yell,
and sit in the stands.
Have you guessed this letter?
Yes, F is for Fans!

Fans come in all shapes and sizes and all different volumes but they have one thing in common: a love for their favourite team!

While NHL arenas sell out on a regular basis, on special occasions, huge numbers of fans have attended hockey games. On December 11, 2010, the University of Michigan Wolverines shut out the Michigan State Spartans 5–0 at Michigan Stadium in Ann Arbor, Michigan, with 104,173 fans watching, setting a Guinness World Record for attendance at a hockey game.

The 2003 Heritage Classic at Commonwealth Stadium in Edmonton set the standard for the number of fans watching an NHL game when 57,167 saw the Montreal Canadiens edge the Edmonton Oilers 4–3.

The record attendance for a Stanley Cup playoff game is 28,183 when the visiting Philadelphia Flyers defeated the hometown Tampa Bay Lightning 4–1 at the Thunderdome.

Fans also love to wear the jerseys of their favourite players. The top-selling jerseys in the 2010–11 season were: 1) Sidney Crosby, Pittsburgh Penguins; 2) Alexander Ovechkin, Washington Capitals; 3) Evgeni Malkin, Pittsburgh Penguins; 4) Marc-Andre Fleury, Pittsburgh Penguins; and 5) Mike Richards, Philadelphia Flyers.

Ff

Goalie is our **G**.
His equipment is thick
for stopping the puck
along with his stick.

Gg

In hockey's earliest days, goalies did not wear much protective equipment. Usually, it was little more than leg pads along with their skates and stick. No trapper, no blocker, and even no mask! But then, back at that time, goalies were not allowed to fall to the ice to block shots. When that rule changed, the need for added protection became more important, and today there is no NHL goalie that plays without a mask, chest protector, arm pads, large leg pads, and special skates.

In the NHL, each year the best goalie is awarded the Vezina Trophy, and the goalies on the team that allow the fewest goals during the regular season receive the William Jennings Trophy.

Before the start of the 1926–27 season, the Montreal Canadiens donated a trophy to the NHL that would be awarded annually to the league's best goaltender. The trophy was the Vezina Trophy, named after Georges Vezina, who died on March 27, 1926. He had been the only goaltender to play for the Montreal Canadiens between 1910 and 1925.

Among the great goalies who have won the Vezina Trophy are Martin Brodeur, Ken Dryden, Dominik Hasek (six times), Jacques Plante (seven times), Patrick Roy, Terry Sawchuk, and Tim Thomas.

The Hockey Hall of Fame began in 1943, even though there was not an actual building. Instead, each year, players were added, and their names reported in newspapers and on the radio. It wasn't until 1961 that the Hall of Fame had a building. It was located in Toronto on the grounds of the Canadian National Exhibition. Today, located in the heart of Toronto's downtown, the Hockey Hall of Fame is home to the largest collection of hockey artifacts anywhere in the world, and it is also home to the Stanley Cup!

For most hockey players, reaching the NHL is a dream from childhood. It is almost too hard to imagine ever being one of the players elected each year to the Hockey Hall of Fame.

Denis Savard, who was inducted into the Hockey Hall of Fame in 2000, stated, "Being elected to the Hockey Hall of Fame is something I'll cherish forever. The Hockey Hall of Fame is the ultimate for any hockey player. It's something that's going to stay there forever. When I have grandkids and they have their own kids, they'll be able to go there and see it. For me, to be part of that is the greatest thrill in sports in my life!"

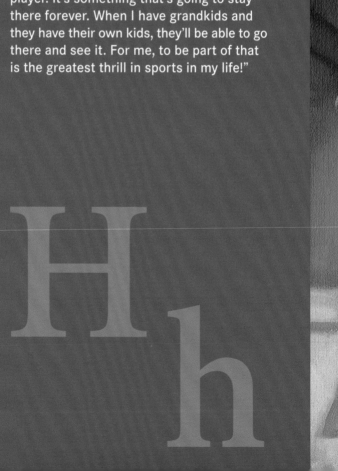

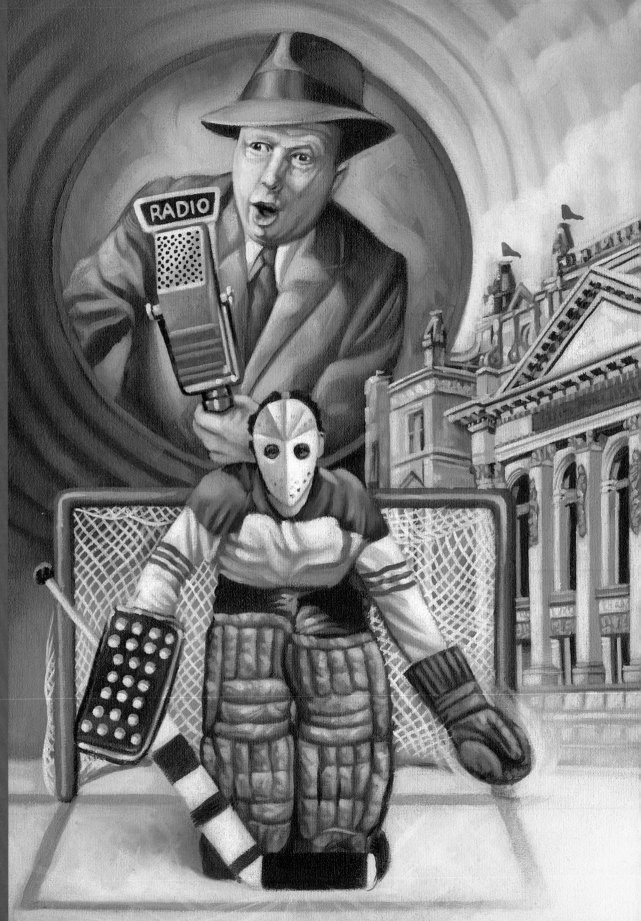

H is for Hockey
and its Hall of Fame.
The wonderful home
of the best in the game.

I i

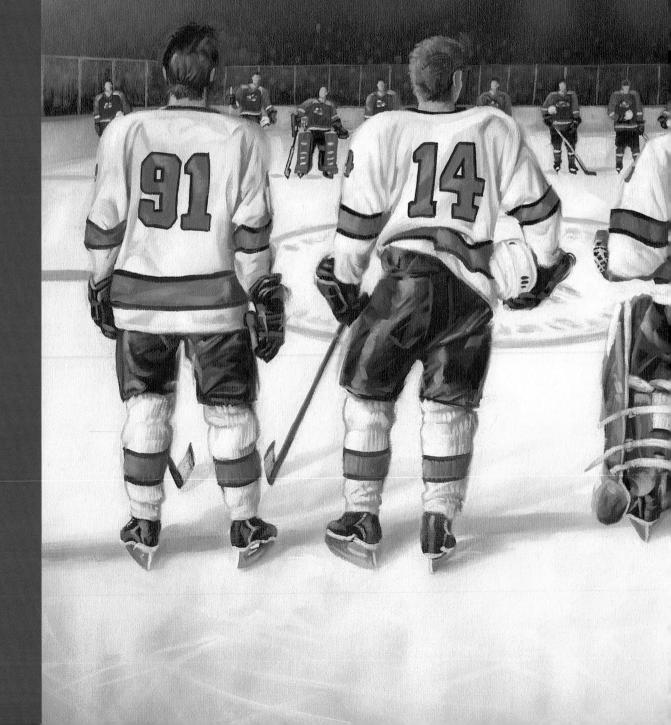

I is for Ice.
It's so cold to the touch.
With a stick and a puck
it's enjoyed oh so much!

Have you heard about the Lucky Loonie? In Canada, there is a one-dollar coin called a "loonie." In 2002, Dan Craig from Edmonton, Alberta was hired to make the ice at the Winter Olympic Games in Salt Lake City, Utah. He did a wonderful job, but while working to make the surface perfect, he buried a loonie in the ice under the centre face-off circle, hoping the coin would bring good luck to his fellow Canadians. It certainly did!

On February 21, Team Canada's women defeated the United States 3–2 to win the gold medal. The team had heard whispers of a "lucky loonie" buried beneath centre ice, and the players, including Cassie Campbell, Jayna Hefford, and Hayley Wickenheiser, crouched around the spot to see the coin. They were hurriedly asked to leave the ice as no one was to know about the secret good luck charm. Three days later, Team Canada's men beat the United States, with Jarome Iginla and Joe Sakic both scoring twice in a 5–2 victory.

The "Lucky Loonie" had worked, as both Team Canada's women and men won Olympic gold medals.

Wayne Gretzky, the executive director of Team Canada's men, carved the coin out of the ice and later presented it to the Hockey Hall of Fame.

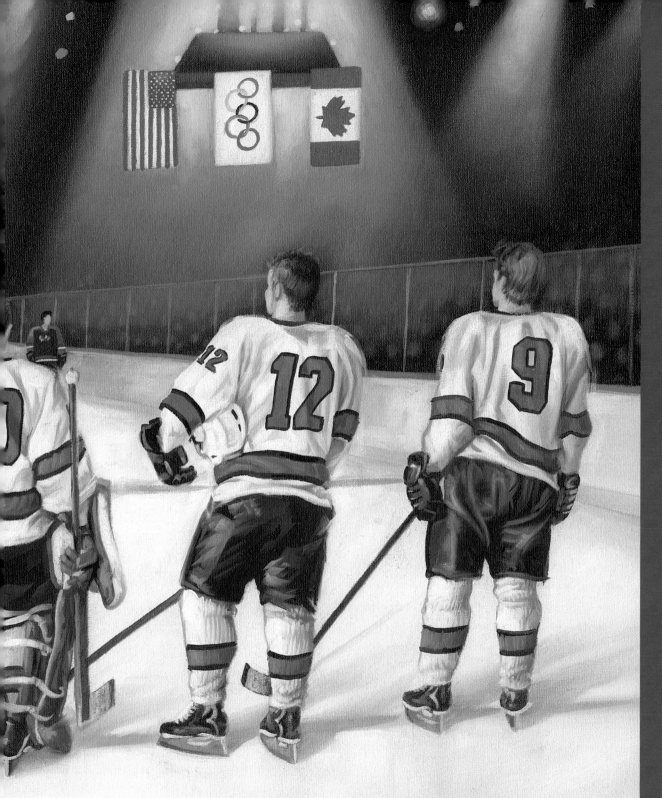

From hockey's humble beginnings, teams wore distinctive jerseys so that players and fans could tell the teams apart. The idea of putting numbers on the backs of jerseys didn't come about until the Pacific Coast Hockey Association (PCHA), which operated from 1912 to 1924, introduced the idea of adding numbers as a way for fans to tell which player was which.

Jersey numbers make for some interesting stories. Jordin Tootoo of the Nashville Predators wears number 22 ("two-two") on the back of his jersey. When Mike Commodore played with the Detroit Red Wings, he wore 64 on his back. Back in the 1980s, many youngsters played computer games on a Commodore 64.

Pulling the jersey of an NHL team over your head fulfills the dreams of many youngsters. Riley Cote, who was a Philadelphia Flyer in 2006–07 and 2009–10, stated, "It was an honour every time to pull that orange-and-black jersey over my head." Ryan VandenBussche, who played nine NHL seasons between the New York Rangers, Chicago Blackhawks, and Pittsburgh Penguins, said, "I'll never forget pulling on an NHL jersey for the first time. It was in New York, and the Rangers just called me up. I remember being in the dressing room at Madison Square Garden, sitting in my stall and putting on my jersey thinking, 'Wow! This is cool!'"

Every player on a team
must dress the same way
so each wears a Jersey—
that word starts with J.

Jj

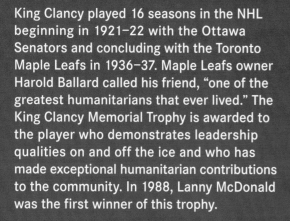

Kk

King Clancy played 16 seasons in the NHL beginning in 1921–22 with the Ottawa Senators and concluding with the Toronto Maple Leafs in 1936–37. Maple Leafs owner Harold Ballard called his friend, "one of the greatest humanitarians that ever lived." The King Clancy Memorial Trophy is awarded to the player who demonstrates leadership qualities on and off the ice and who has made exceptional humanitarian contributions to the community. In 1988, Lanny McDonald was the first winner of this trophy.

There are several trophies that awarded annually honour former NHL players:

Bill Masterton Memorial Trophy: Masterton died during an NHL game in 1968. This trophy is given annually for perseverance, sportsmanship, and dedication to hockey.

Jack Adams Award: presented to the NHL coach who has contributed the most to his team's success. The trophy honours the coaching career of Jack Adams.

Vezina Trophy: honours Georges Vezina, who died of tuberculosis after collapsing during a game in 1925. The Vezina Trophy goes to the NHL's best goalkeeper.

Maurice "Rocket" Richard Trophy: donated by the Montreal Canadiens. Richard spent his entire 18-season career with the Canadiens. This trophy is presented to the NHL's regular season goal-scoring leader.

Ted Lindsay Award: honours Lindsay's skill and tenacity, as well as the leadership role he took in establishing the original Players' Association. This award is presented to the most outstanding player during the NHL's regular season.

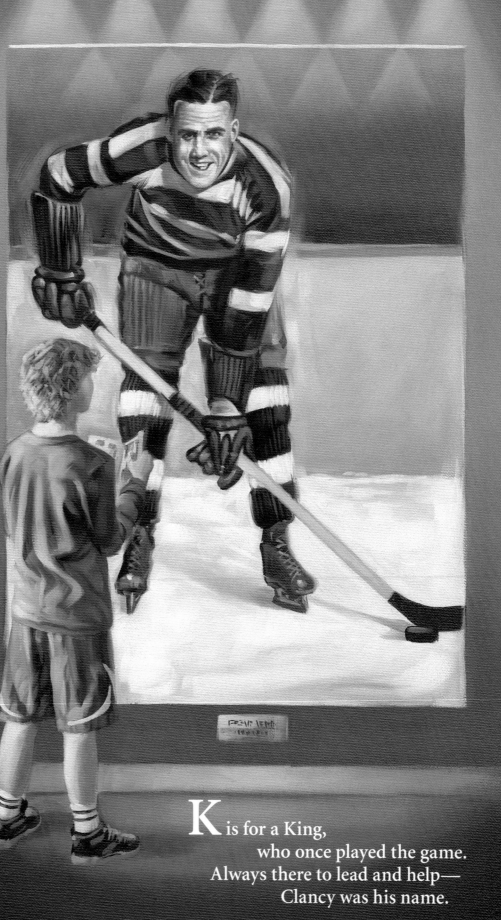

K is for a King,
who once played the game.
Always there to lead and help—
Clancy was his name.

Ted Lindsay's outstanding NHL career lasted 17 seasons. During that time, he was an All-Star nine times, the NHL's leading scorer once, and was a member of four Stanley Cup championships. An Honoured Member of the Hockey Hall of Fame, Ted Lindsay's greatest contribution to hockey away from the ice may very well be his initiation of an association for players to help them earn better salaries and pensions for their retirement. It would take 10 years before this player's association would take hold in the National Hockey League.

Today, the most valuable player during the regular season, voted on by the players, is awarded the Ted Lindsay Award.

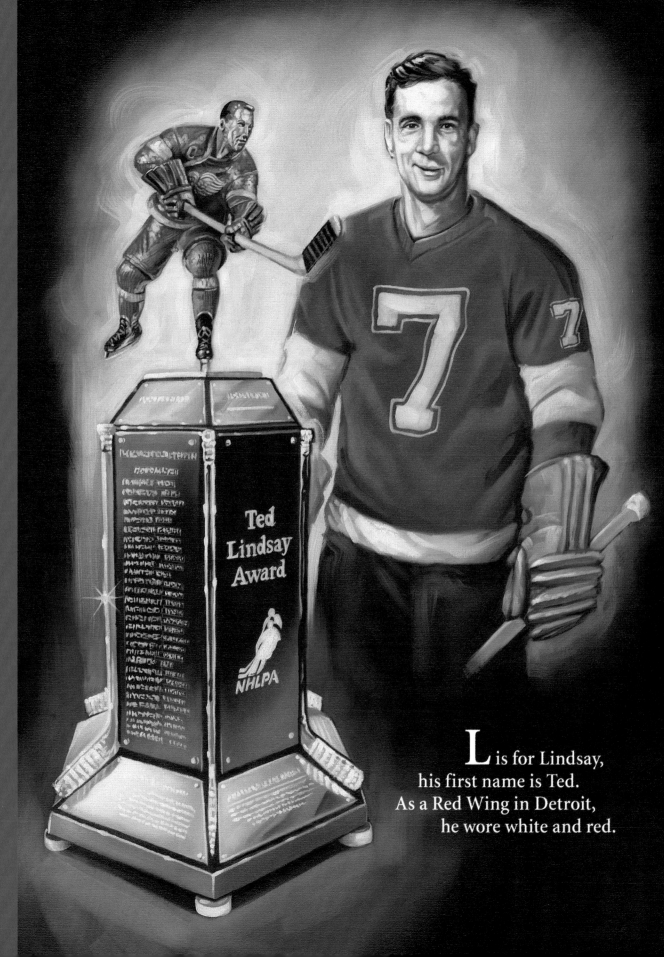

L is for Lindsay,
his first name is Ted.
As a Red Wing in Detroit,
he wore white and red.

A top sports moment—
you may know this story.
M is the Miracle
of this team's gold medal glory.

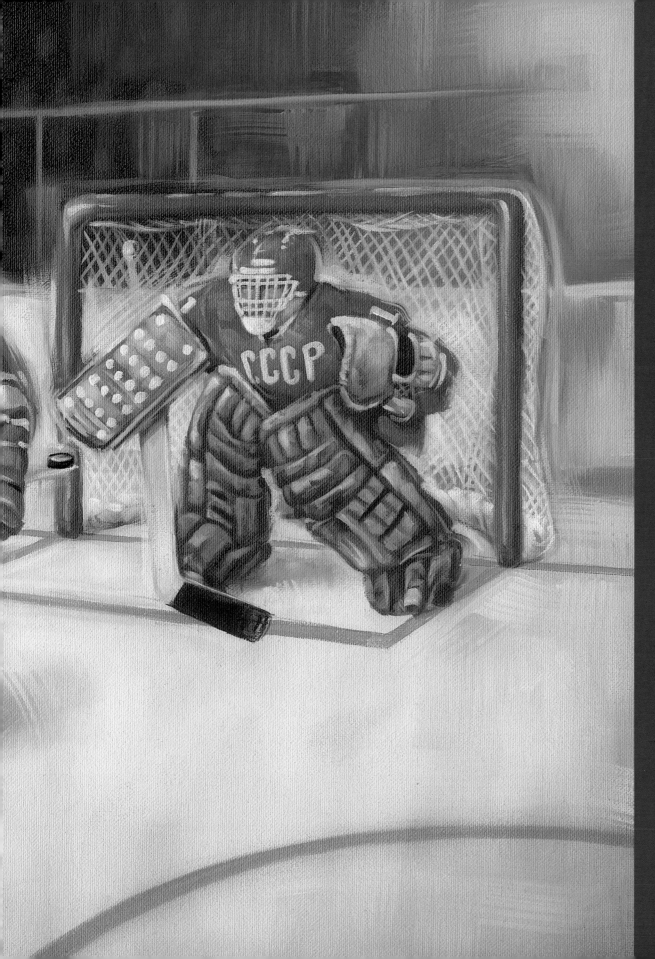

In 1980, the Olympic Winter Games were held in Lake Placid, New York. The Olympic men's hockey team for the United States wasn't given much chance of winning.

At that time, professional players were not allowed to participate in the Olympics, so Team USA was stocked with young college hockey players. The team, fired up by their coach, shocked the hockey world by defeating the powerful Soviet team, and then Finland, to win the gold medal.

Team USA's victory was so unlikely that it was called the "Miracle on Ice." In 1999, *Sports Illustrated* magazine selected the "Miracle on Ice" as the top sports moment of the twentieth century!

Thirteen members of Team USA went on to NHL careers. Goaltenders Jim Craig and Steve Janaszak, defencemen Bill Baker, Dave Christian, Ken Morrow (who was part of four Stanley Cup championships with the New York Islanders), Jack O'Callahan, and Mike Ramsey as well as forwards Neil Broten (a member of the New Jersey Devils when they won the Stanley Cup in 1995), Steve Christoff, Mark Johnson, Rob McClanahan, Mark Pavelich, and Dave Silk all went on to play in the NHL. Coach Herb Brooks later coached four NHL teams.

There have been two films made about this team: *Miracle on Ice* in 1981 and *Miracle* in 2004.

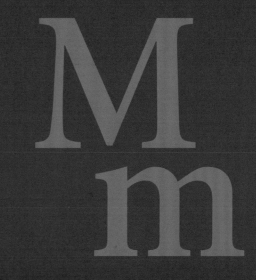

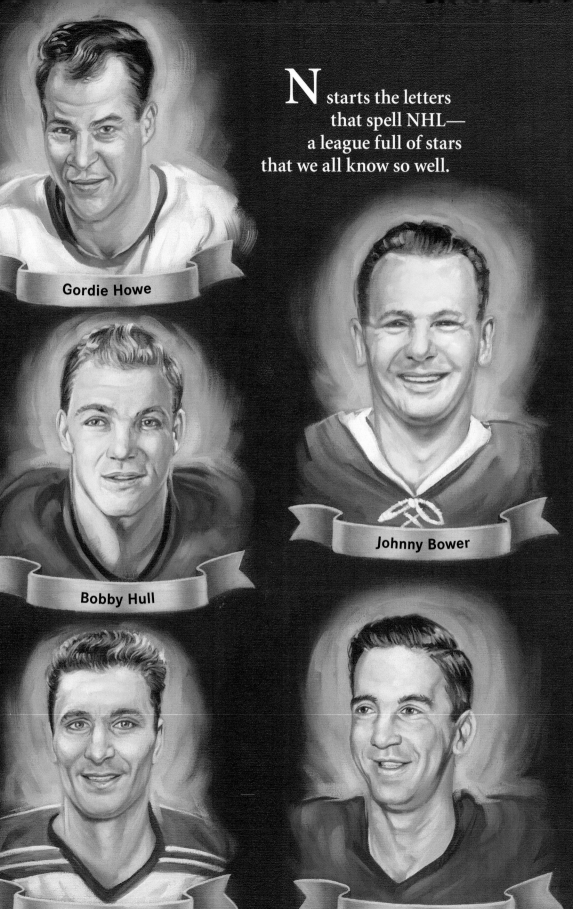

N starts the letters
that spell NHL—
a league full of stars
that we all know so well.

Gordie Howe

Bobby Hull

Johnny Bower

Andy Bathgate

Ted Lindsay

The National Hockey League, known as the NHL, is the premier professional hockey league in the world.

The NHL was created on November 22, 1917 in Montreal after the suspension of a previous league called the National Hockey Association (NHA). The NHL began with four teams, although one had to leave the league after six games when its arena burned down.

Today, the NHL is proudly made up of 30 teams spread throughout the United States and Canada. There are seven NHL teams in Canada (Calgary Flames, Edmonton Oilers, Montreal Canadiens, Ottawa Senators, Toronto Maple Leafs, Vancouver Canucks, and Winnipeg Jets) and 23 from the United States (Anaheim Ducks, Boston Bruins, Buffalo Sabres, Carolina Hurricanes, Chicago Blackhawks, Colorado Avalanche, Columbus Blue Jackets, Dallas Stars, Detroit Red Wings, Los Angeles Kings, Minnesota Wild, Florida Panthers, Nashville Predators, New Jersey Devils, New York Islanders, New York Rangers, Philadelphia Flyers, Phoenix Coyotes, Pittsburgh Penguins, San Jose Sharks, St. Louis Blues, Tampa Bay Lightning, and Washington Capitals).

Each team plays an 82–game season that decides which teams participate in the playoffs. And each spring, one team wins the NHL's championship trophy—the Stanley Cup!

N n

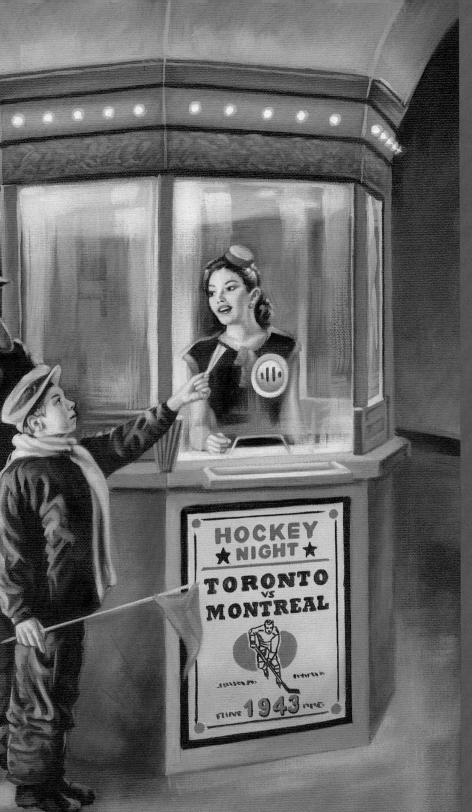

Original Six
starts with an **O**.
These first NHL teams
helped to make the league grow.

Even though the NHL has an Original Six, the league actually began with just four teams when it was formed in 1917—the Montreal Canadiens, Montreal Wanderers (who withdrew after six games), Ottawa Senators, and Toronto Hockey Club. The league operated with just three teams in 1918–19 and then, for the next 25 years, the league expanded and contracted to include such long-forgotten teams as the Hamilton Tigers, Montreal Maroons, New York Americans, Philadelphia Quakers, Pittsburgh Pirates, Quebec Bulldogs, and the St. Louis Eagles.

It wasn't until 1942–43 that the NHL had six teams: the Boston Bruins, Chicago Black Hawks, Detroit Red Wings, Montreal Canadiens, New York Rangers, and the Toronto Maple Leafs. The Chicago team was Black Hawks (two words) until the 1980s when they changed to Blackhawks.

The NHL was made up of those six teams for 25 years, and that period of time is known as the Original Six era. It is considered to be hockey's greatest era. In 1967–68, the NHL added six more teams, ending the Original Six era. Today, there are 30 teams competing in the league.

Each NHL team plays 82 games during the regular season. The winner of the Western Conference then faces the winner of the Eastern Conference, and the team that wins the best-of-seven series wins the NHL's greatest prize—the Stanley Cup!

There have been sensational playoff moments through the years. Bill Barilko of the Toronto Maple Leafs scored the Stanley Cup–winning goal for Toronto against Montreal in 1951 and then, later that summer, he died in a plane crash, and his body was not found for 11 years.

On April 23, 1964, Bob Baun of the Maple Leafs broke his ankle during the third period of a playoff game against the Detroit Red Wings. After having it frozen and taped, he returned to the game and scored the winning goal at 1:43 of overtime! The win tied the series at three wins apiece, and allowed Toronto to win the Stanley Cup in Game 7.

Bobby Orr of the Boston Bruins scored the Stanley Cup–winning goal in overtime in 1970 while flying through the air after being tripped by a St. Louis Blues defenceman.

The longest Stanley Cup playoff ever ended when Modere "Mud" Bruneteau of the Detroit Red Wings scored at 16:30 of the sixth overtime period on March 24, 1936, to give his team a 1–0 win over the Montreal Maroons. That is almost three complete games played back-to-back!

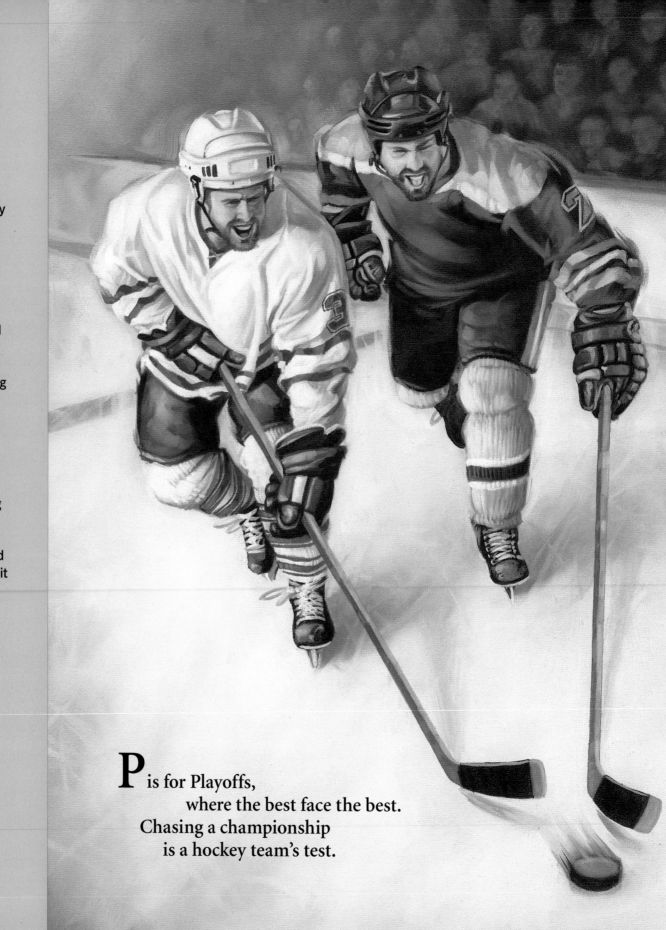

P is for Playoffs,
where the best face the best.
Chasing a championship
is a hockey team's test.

The NHL was created on November 22, 1917, in Montreal, Quebec.

Today, after several expansions and with teams moving to new cities, there are 30 teams in the NHL, spread across North America.

The Montreal Canadiens are the only team that has been in the league since the very beginning. The franchise has also won more Stanley Cup championships than any other team—24!

But the Montreal Canadiens aren't the only NHL team that has come from Quebec. There were the Montreal Wanderers from the 1917–18 season, the Montreal Maroons from 1924–25 to 1937–38, the Quebec Bulldogs, who played in the NHL during the 1919–20 season, and the Quebec Nordiques, which was a member club of the NHL from 1972–73 to 1994–95.

Players from the province of Quebec who have excelled in the NHL through the years include Jean Béliveau, Martin Brodeur, Marcel Dionne, Dave Keon, Guy Lafleur, Maurice Richard, Luc Robitaille, and Gump Worsley.

Qq

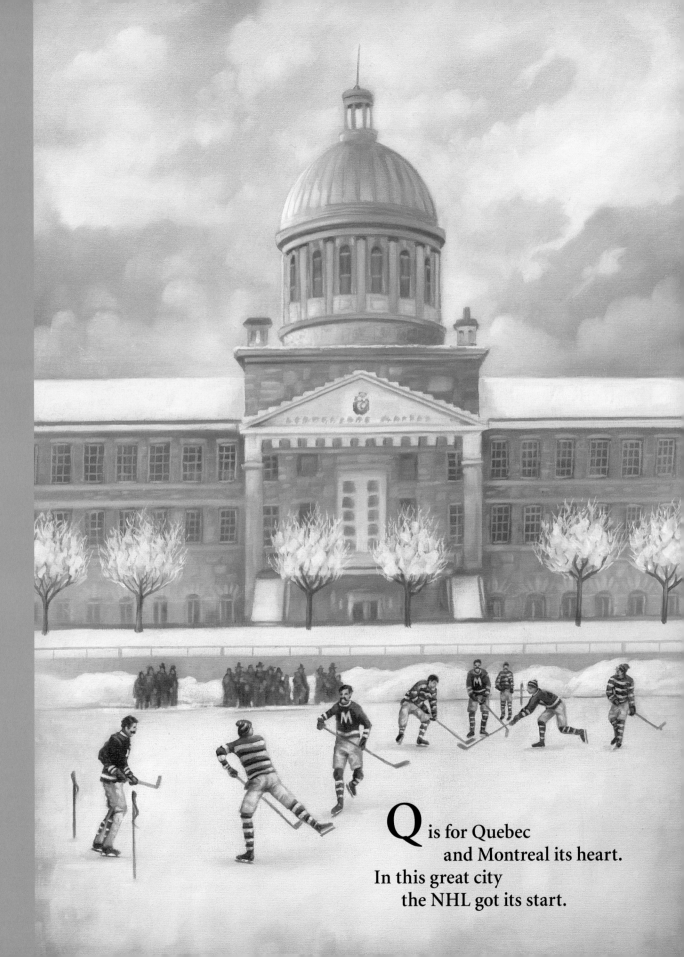

Q is for Quebec
        and Montreal its heart.
In this great city
        the NHL got its start.

Rr

When a team retires a number to honour a former player, that number is not worn again by anyone who plays on that team afterwards.

The first retired number came from the Toronto Maple Leafs in 1934 to honour Irvine "Ace" Bailey, who was injured in a game and was never able to play again. His jersey number 6 was retired, never to be worn by another Maple Leaf. That began a tradition of teams retiring jersey numbers. Since then most teams have retired at least one player's number, some because the player was such a star that they wanted to acknowledge his contributions and other times because a tragedy occurred and it was a way for the team to honour the player's memory.

The Montreal Canadiens have retired 17 jersey numbers, the most of any team.

Only one jersey has been retired across the entire NHL. After a phenomenal career, the NHL retired Wayne Gretzky's 99 on February 6, 2000. No NHL player will ever wear that number again.

When the Minnesota Wild joined the NHL in 2000, they retired the number 1 as a tribute to their fans!

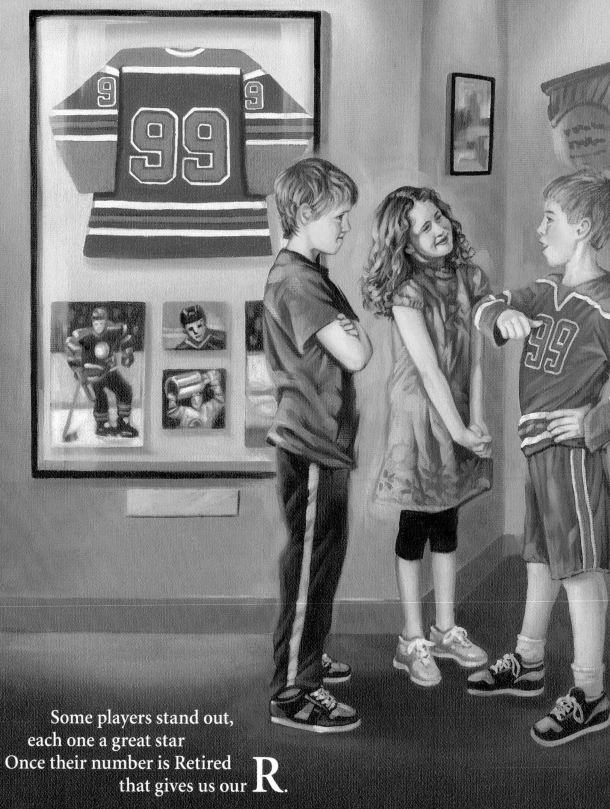

"THE GREAT ONE"

Some players stand out,
each one a great star
Once their number is Retired
that gives us our **R**.

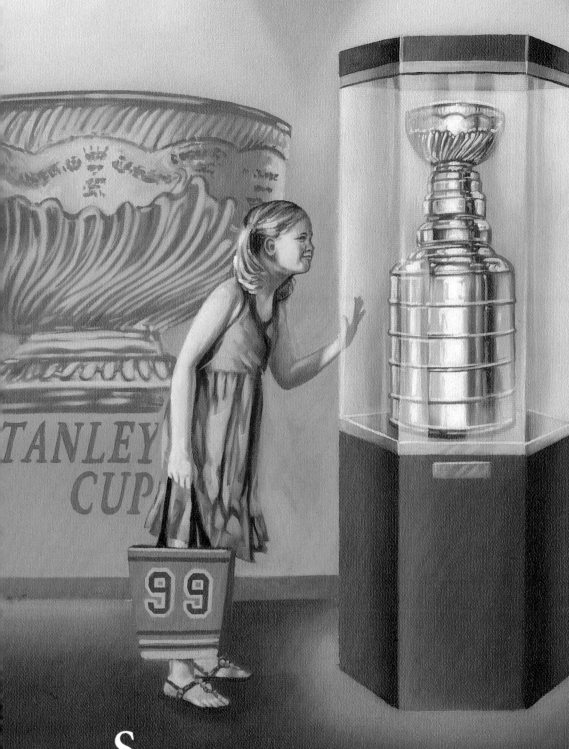

S stands for Stanley
and a Cup that's so great.
Named for a governor general
who never could skate!

Queen Victoria appointed Lord Frederick Arthur Stanley as Canada's sixth governor general. He and his family moved from England to Canada to assume his new position in 1888, staying until 1893.

Although the sport of hockey was new to the Stanley family, they embraced it immediately. Lord Stanley's sons formed a team that played games throughout Ontario and helped popularize the sport. His daughter Isobel also loved the game and put together the first known women's team.

In 1892, Lord Stanley donated a trophy to be awarded each year to the best amateur hockey team in Canada. Although originally engraved as the Dominion Hockey Challenge Cup, we know that same trophy today as the Stanley Cup.

Through hockey's growth, the Stanley Cup has changed in many ways. It is now awarded to the best professional hockey team in the NHL. But Lord Stanley's original bowl, which was 7¼ inches (18.5 cm) tall, has been replaced by the version we see awarded today, which is 35¼ inches (89.54 cm) in height.

By the way, Lord Stanley never got to see the trophy he donated awarded to a winning team. He and his family returned to England in 1893 before the Montreal Hockey Club from the Montreal Amateur Athletic Association was presented with the trophy as the first Stanley Cup champions.

Ss

Tt

Three Stars are selected
at the end of each game.
They skate out for the fans
when they announce each one's name.

The Three Stars selection at the conclusion of each game is a popular and longstanding tradition in hockey, honouring the three best players in that contest.

The practice began in 1936–37 as a way for Imperial Oil (now known as Esso) to advertise its Imperial Three Star brand of gasoline on *Hockey Night in Canada* radio broadcasts. Although that brand of gasoline is long gone, the tradition continues today and is a common practice in all NHL arenas.

On March 23, 1944, Maurice "Rocket" Richard scored all five goals in the Montreal Canadiens' playoff win over the Toronto Maple Leafs, and for his terrific play, he was named all three stars!

After Wayne Gretzky played his final NHL game when the New York Rangers faced the Pittsburgh Penguins on April 18, 1999, Gretzky was also awarded all three stars, honouring his contributions to hockey throughout an exceptional career.

The NHL began in 1917 but it took until 1924 for the first American team to join the league. That year, Charles Adams, who owned a chain of grocery stores, was granted an NHL team. He asked his general manager, Art Ross, to choose a nickname that would reflect a wild animal that possessed quickness and intellect. Ross selected *bruin*, an old English word for a brown bear.

Boston was already a good hockey town with several amateur teams, so fans immediately began attending games played at home by this new team ... even though they won only six games in their first season. But clever player acquisitions soon made the team very competitive. The Bruins won the Stanley Cup in just their fifth season.

The Boston Bruins have captured the Stanley Cup on six occasions: 1929, 1939, 1941, 1970, 1972, and 2011.

Ten Bruins have had their jersey numbers retired by the franchise. Eddie Shore's number 2, Lionel Hitchman's number 3, Bobby Orr's number 4, Dit Clapper's number 5, Phil Esposito's number 7, Cam Neely's number 8, Johnny Bucyk's number 9, Milt Schmidt's number 15, Terry O'Reilly's number 24, and Ray Bourque's number 77 all hang from the rafters of the TD Garden in Boston.

U u

The first NHL team from the United States was the Bruins from Boston, one of the league's early greats.

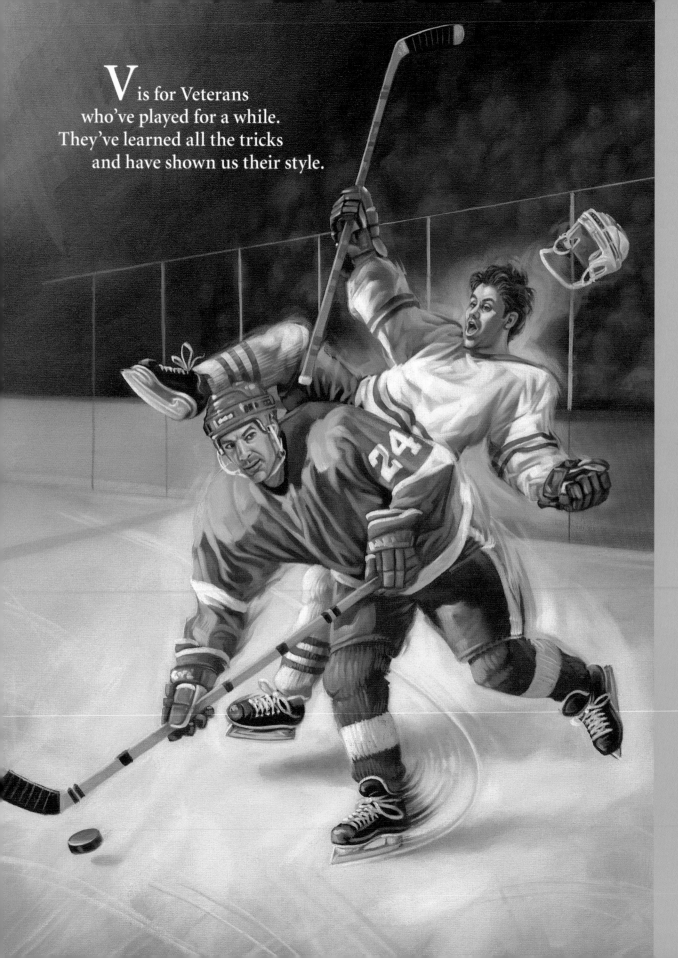

V is for Veterans
who've played for a while.
They've learned all the tricks
and have shown us their style.

The oldest player to play in the NHL was Gordie Howe, who retired in 1980 when he was 52 years old! Gordie played 26 seasons in the NHL—25 with the Detroit Red Wings and one with the Hartford Whalers.

Chris Chelios is an NHL veteran who played 26 seasons for the Montreal Canadiens, Chicago Blackhawks, Detroit Red Wings, and Atlanta Thrashers before retiring in 2010 at the age of 48. He was the second oldest player ever to play in the NHL.

There are five Hall of Famers who played in the NHL at an advanced age. Johnny Bower was 45 when he retired, and Doug Harvey, Tim Horton, Jacques Plante, and Gump Worsley were all 44.

On November 25, 1951, Chicago's goalie, Harry Lumley, was injured in a game. There were no replacement goalies at that time, so the job fell to the Black Hawks' assistant trainer, Moe Roberts, a retired goalie. Two weeks shy of his 46th birthday, Roberts played the last period of the game, shutting out the Red Wings, but the Hawks lost 5–2. It was his final action in the NHL.

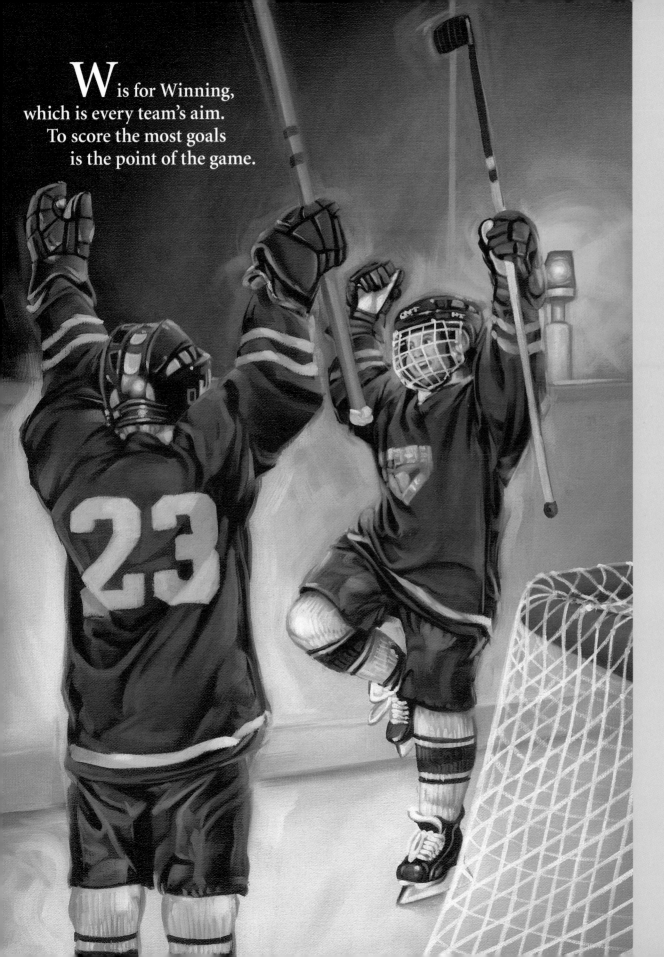

W is for Winning,
which is every team's aim.
To score the most goals
is the point of the game.

The idea behind hockey is, of course, to win. And to win, you must score more goals than your opponent.

In 1995–96, the Detroit Red Wings set an NHL record for most wins in one season when they won 62 games. In 1992–93, the Pittsburgh Penguins established a record by winning 17 games in a row.

The most goals scored by one team in an NHL game was 16. On March 3, 1920, the Montreal Canadiens defeated the Quebec Bulldogs 16–3. That same season, the Canadiens also set the record for most goals scored by two teams in a single game when they combined with the Toronto St. Pats on January 10, 1920 to collect 21 goals, with Montreal winning 14–7. That record was tied by the Edmonton Oilers and Chicago Blackhawks on December 11, 1985 when the Oilers won 12–9.

On March 23, 1952, in the final regular season game for the Chicago Black Hawks and New York Rangers, two records were set simultaneously as Chicago edged the Rangers 7–6. In that game, Bill Mosienko of the Black Hawks scored the fastest three goals in NHL history. He scored his hat trick within 21 seconds. Gus Bodnar set the record for the fastest three assists when he contributed to each of Mosienko's goals.

W
W

X x

From its beginning in 1917, the NHL has grown from four teams, has been reduced to just three, and now has grown to have 30 amazing teams from around the United States and Canada, all challenging one another for the Stanley Cup.

Canada's western-most team is in Vancouver, with two Alberta-based teams (Calgary and Edmonton), one in Winnipeg, Manitoba, both the Toronto Maple Leafs and Ottawa Senators in Ontario and the Montreal Canadiens in Quebec.

There are 23 teams from the United States, spanning 17 states. California and New York each have three teams. The Anaheim Ducks, Los Angeles Kings, and San Jose Sharks are based in California while New York State has the Buffalo Sabres, New York Islanders, and New York Rangers.

Florida has two teams (the Panthers, who play in Miami, and the Lightning from Tampa) as does Pennsylvania with the Philadelphia Flyers and Pittsburgh Penguins. The remaining 13 states are Arizona (Phoenix Coyotes), Carolina (Hurricanes), Colorado (The Avalanche), Illinois (Chicago Blackhawks), Massachusetts (Boston Bruins), Michigan (Detroit Red Wings), Minnesota (The Wild), Missouri (St. Louis Blues), New Jersey (Devils), Ohio (Columbus Blue Jackets), Tennessee (Nashville Predators), Texas (Dallas Stars) and Washington, D.C. (Capitals).

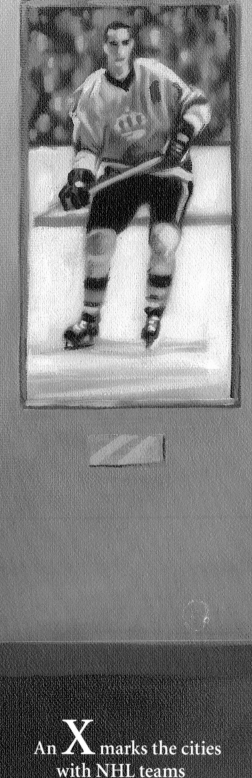

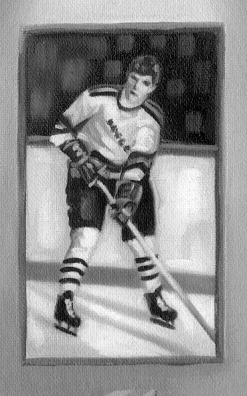

An **X** marks the cities
with NHL teams
where the greatest of players
chase Stanley Cup dreams.

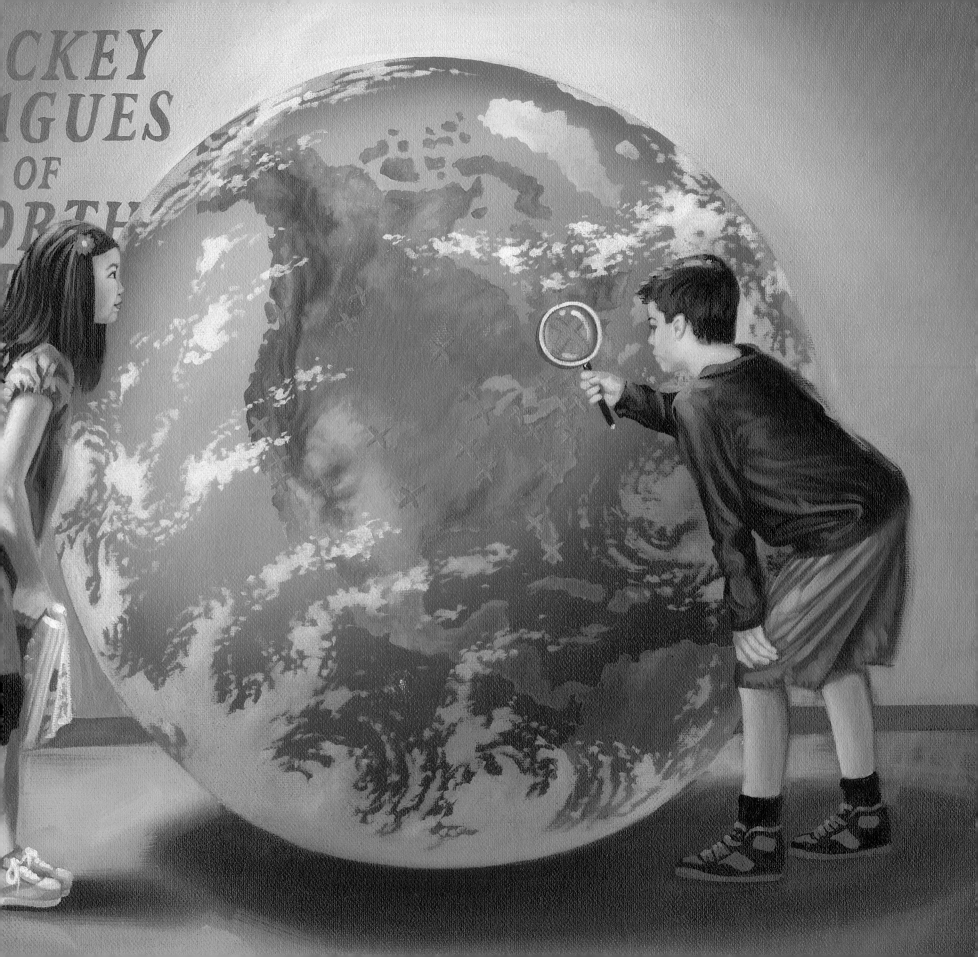

In January 1905, the Dawson City Nuggets, made up mostly of miners from Dawson City in Canada's Yukon Territory, challenged the Ottawa Silver Seven for the Stanley Cup championship.

At the time, there were no airplanes, so the Dawson City players travelled by dogsled and bicycle to Whitehorse. They then boarded a train to Skagway, Alaska where they met a ship that took them to Vancouver, British Columbia. A cross-country train made the trek across the country to Ottawa so that the Nuggets could challenge the reigning Stanley Cup champion Ottawa Silver Seven. The trip covered 4,000 miles (6,400 km) and took one month to complete.

In the first game, played on January 13, 1905, Ottawa beat Dawson City 9–2. Three days later, the Ottawa Silver Seven blasted the Dawson City Nuggets 23–2. Frank McGee, the star of the Silver Seven, scored 14 goals. The unfortunate Dawson City goalie was 17-year-old Albert Forrest.

The series was to have been a best-of-five, but both teams agreed that there was no need to play any further games. The Stanley Cup was awarded to Ottawa again.

Y is for Yukon
and its Stanley Cup quest.
Took train, ship, and dogsled
to challenge the best.

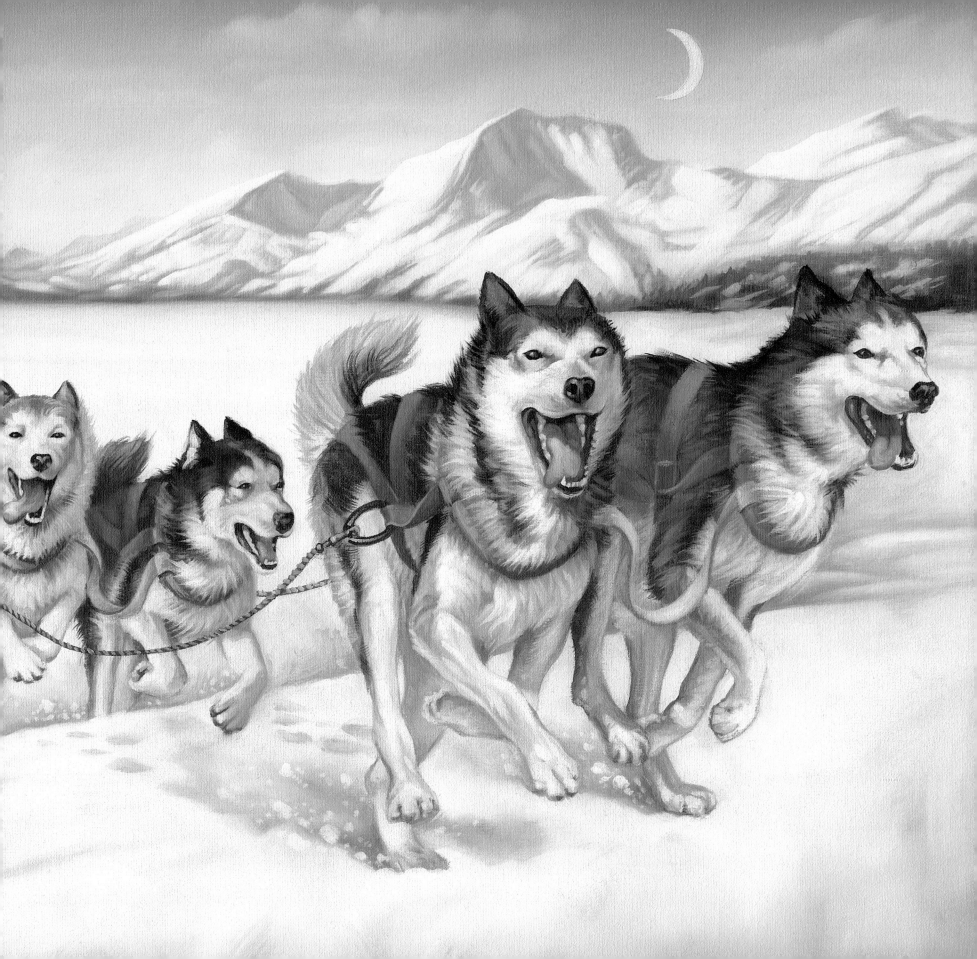

Any goalie will tell you that it takes skill, luck, and a total team effort in order to record a shutout. But it is the netminder who is credited with the shutout when his team allows zero goals.

George Hainsworth, a goalie with the Montreal Canadiens, recorded 22 shutouts in 1928–29, and teams only played 44 games in a season at that time!

Terry Sawchuk recorded his first shutout with the Detroit Red Wings in 1949–50 and his 103rd while playing with the New York Rangers in 1969–70. When he hit the 100-shutout plateau on March 4, 1967, Sawchuk was a member of the Toronto Maple Leafs. He was named First Star of the game and afterwards, shook the hands of each of his teammates. "The ovation from the Toronto fans is something I'll never forget," he said.

Hockey fans believed that Sawchuk's record would never be broken, but along came Martin Brodeur of the New Jersey Devils. On December 21, 2009, Martin earned his 104th regular season shutout to set the new NHL shutout record. "When you do break records and you see how long they've lasted, it's pretty cool," he said. "It's a great honour for me to be in that position."

Z z

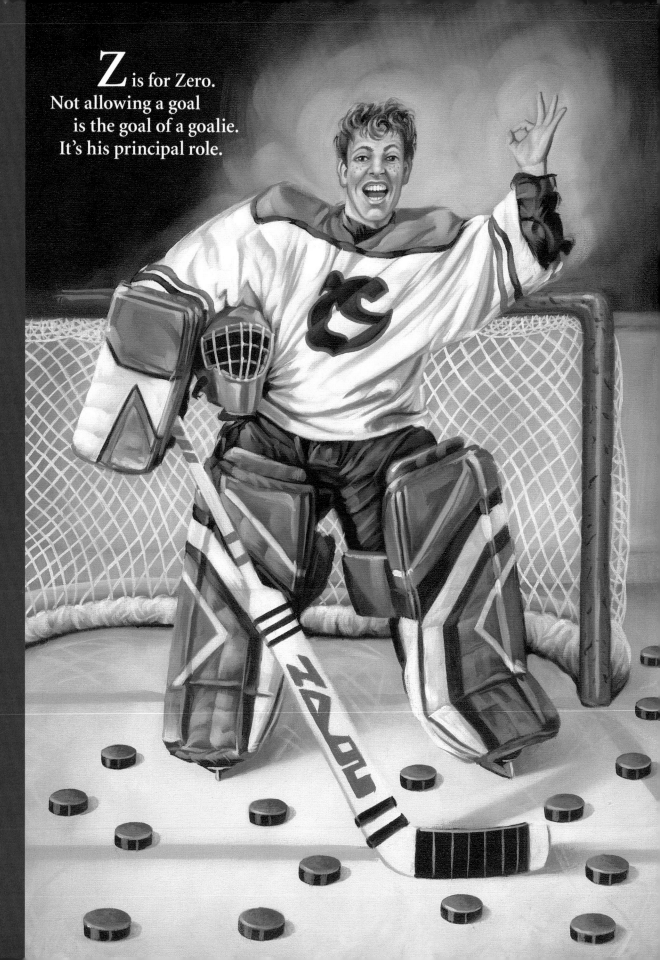

Z is for Zero.
Not allowing a goal
is the goal of a goalie.
It's his principal role.